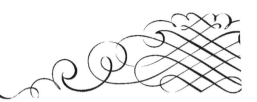
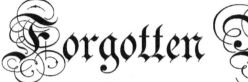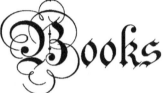
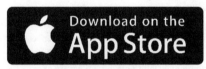
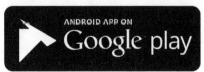

ISBN 978-1-334-97944-6
PIBN 10783626

This book is a reproduction of an important historical work. Forgotten Books uses
state-of-the-art technology to digitally reconstruct the work, preserving the original format
whilst repairing imperfections present in the aged copy. In rare cases, an imperfection in
the original, such as a blemish or missing page, may be replicated in our edition. We do,
however, repair the vast majority of imperfections successfully; any imperfections that
remain are intentionally left to preserve the state of such historical works.

1 MONTH OF
FREE
READING

at

www.ForgottenBooks.com

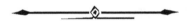

By purchasing this book you are eligible for one month membership to ForgottenBooks.com, giving you unlimited access to our entire collection of over 700,000 titles via our web site and mobilc apps.

To claim your free month visit:

www.forgottenbooks.com/free783626

English
Français
Deutsche
Italiano
Español
Português

www.forgottenbooks.com

Mythology Photography **Fiction**
Fishing Christianity **Art** Cooking
Essays Buddhism Freemasonry
Medicine **Biology** Music **Ancient
Egypt** Evolution Carpentry Physics
Dance Geology **Mathematics** Fitness
Shakespeare **Folklore** Yoga Marketing
Confidence Immortality Biographies
Poetry **Psychology** Witchcraft
Electronics Chemistry History **Law**
Accounting **Philosophy** Anthropology
Alchemy Drama Quantum Mechanics
Atheism Sexual Health **Ancient History**
Entrepreneurship Languages Sport
Paleontology Needlework Islam
Metaphysics Investment Archaeology
Parenting Statistics Criminology
Motivational

THE

HEALTH AND DISEASES

—— OF ——

WOMAN

BY

R. T. TRALL, M. D.

Author of the "Hydropathic Encyclopedia;" "Hygienic Hand Book;"
"Uterine Diseases and Displacements;" "The True Healing
Art;" "True Temperance Platform; "Hygienic
System;" "Tobacco Using;" &c., &c.

———— ✦ ————

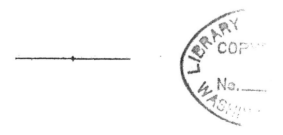

PUBLISHED AT
THE OFFICE OF THE HEALTH REFORMER,
BATTLE CREEK, MICH.
1873.

PREFACE.

TEN years ago, an edition of 5000 copies of this work was published in New York, and rapidly sold, since which time it has been out of print. But it has been so often called for, and seems, moreover, to be one of the desiderata of the Hygienic literature of the day, that I have concluded to revise it, and have it republished. I have made some important additions, and have corroborated the statements of the author by some pungent, and, I trust, instructive quotations from the latest medical authors on the subject of the diseases of women, and of the pernicious habits and fashionable follies which conduce to them.

R. T. TRALL, M. D.

Florence Hights, N. J., Oct. 25, 1872.

TESTIMONIAL.

HAVING carefully examined the following pages treating upon the important subject of health and diseases of woman, we bear cheerful testimony to its merits, believing it surpasses any work of the kind ever placed before the public. It points out in a clear, forcible manner the causes that are undermining the health of American women, and shows the terrible effects produced thereby upon their offspring. It portrays to young and old the sad consequences of following wrong habits of life, and the untold miseries resulting from drug medication as sustained by the highest acknowledged medical authority. We therefore unhesitatingly recommend it to every intelligent person in the land. No family should be without it, as it will prove an invaluable help in guiding the household in the paths of virtue and health.

MRS. M. A. CHAMBERLAIN, M. D,
MISS P. M. LAMSON, M. D.

Physicians Health Institute, Battle Creek, Mich.

CONTENTS.

———◆———

HEALTH AND DISEASES OF WOMAN.

WOMAN AND THE MEDICAL PROFESSION.

THE declining health of American women, and the rapidly increasing frailty of American girls, have now become prominent topics of the magazines and newspapers, as well as of the medical journals of the day. And the diseases of woman have long been recognized as the *opprobrium medicorum* of the profession—the disgrace of medical science.

This cannot be because physicians have not had sufficient experience in their treatment; for, in all ages, medical men have had much more to do with the diseases of women than of men; and in this age, and in this country, more than three-fourths of all the practice of the profession are devoted to the treatment of diseases peculiar to women.

At a festival lately held by a medical society in the city of New York, "dear woman" was toasted in the following words: "The last best gift of God to man, and *the chief support of the doctors.*" Do you imagine that when these jovial doctors were feasting themselves full and drinking themselves merry with the avails of this delightful support, they were also devising ways and means to render her healthy, so that she would cease to be the "chief support of the doctors ?"

There are in the United States seventy-five thousand physicians, whose aggregate incomes cannot be less than two hundred millions of dollars; three-fourths of this sum—one hundred and fifty millions—our physicians must thank frail woman for; can they not well afford to compliment her in the ruby wine ?

How can the doctors afford to have the women healthy ? Suppose the women of our country should become reasonably hygienic in their habits of living and in their ways of doctoring, what would be the inevitable result to the profession ? Who cannot see at a glance that more than fifty thousand physicians would be at once thrown out of employment, and half as many drug shops closed for want of customers ? And then there would be the total loss of all the capital and time they had invested in the business and in their education. And, moreover, three-quarters of all the medical schools in the country would be useless, involving a loss of a few millions more.

But the chapter of calamities would not end here; if the women should become generally healthy themselves (for they would not do this without being educated into a knowledge of the conditions of health), they would so arrange their households—their tables, their clothing, their sleeping apartments, and personal habits, that their brothers, husbands, and sons, would have much less occasion to patronize the profession, and so three-fourths of the remaining one-fourth of the medical profession would be liable to lose all they had invested in business, and subjected to the inconveniences of learning a new vocation.

Can the medical profession afford to teach women to be healthy? Shall they make this immense sacrifice for her sake, and for humanity's sake? Is it not asking a little too much of poor human nature? True, it would be a glorious thing for the world; but the world would pay nothing for it—hardly a thank you—while it pays willingly and cheerfully its millions annually to have the women dosed, drugged, poisoned, deceived, miseducated, maltreated, and ruined.

OPIUM—ALCOHOL—TOBACCO—DRUGS.

The British statesmen some years ago discovered that the opium trade, which they have forced on China at the point of the bayonet, was rapidly demoralizing and destroying the people of that nation. And it was suggested in their parliamentary discussions, that motives of justice, and equity, and humanity, and Christianity, demanded its suppression. But what answered the government ? "True enough, it is all wrong and ruinous; it is very bad for the Chinese, but we derive a revenue of twenty millions a year from it; we have got accustomed to this income, and cannot very conveniently dispense with it. Besides, our merchants have invested much money in ships to carry on this commerce." So the opium trade went on.

And the liquor trade, and the tobacco trade, in this country, are practiced on precisely the same principles. The moral sense of all mankind, the intelligent judgment of all the earth, the experience of all the ages, the teachings of science, and the declarations of the Bible, declare those traffics to be abominable and murderous. But the nation derives a revenue from them; our people have invested millions of dollars in these branches of business, and many of them have learned no other vocation, and can see no other way so convenient to earn bread or amass wealth; and so, notwithstanding it is patent to all that these infernal branches of commerce are fast ruining all the nations of the earth, and threatening the total destruction of the human race, the municipal authorities of our cities, the legislatures of our States, and the Congress of our nation, say these traffics must go on. And thus governments, whose legitimate business is to *protect* persons and property, foster, encourage, license, and protect, a business which enables and which authorizes one class of their people to deprave and ruin all the others.

Shall we place the drug trade with the opium trade, the liquor trade, and the tobacco trade? Why not? It is certainly not the least of the four evils; and so far as fraud, and adulteration, and swindling, and killing, are concerned, it outdoes all of them.

Why should doctors and apothecaries be asked to relinquish a profitable business, just because it is injurious to society? Opium-dealers will not do it; rumsellers will not do it; tobacconists will not do it; and why should drug-dealers be expected to do it?

No, no. You, who get gold in the ruin of your fellow-beings, do not expect, you have no right to expect, that physicians will be disinterested, and benevolent, and self-sacrificing, in their dealings with you, until you become at least just in your dealings with others.

I say that to teach our women to be healthy, is to ruin the whole medical profession. So soon as this is done, there will not be a doctor in all the land except the woman physician and the man surgeon.

THE RACE IMPERILED.

The health of woman presents to us another most important consideration. The salvation of the human race absolutely depends upon it. She has to develop the germ of life. It is her function to sustain, nourish, train, and educate, the future man. To a very great extent, she imparts her organic constitution, and stamps her normal or morbid conditions on her offspring. If she is unsound, her children cannot possibly be healthy.

RIGHTS OF OFFSPRING.

And has the offspring no claims—no rights? Let me say to mothers, and let me repeat with still greater emphasis to fathers—for, after all, fathers are more to be blamed in this respect—that every child that is born into the world is entitled to receive, of its earthly parents, the inheritance of a sound organization. Yet, in the present state of society, this is the rare exception instead of the rule. There is no greater sin, there can be no greater crime in all of God's universe, judged by the principle of eternal justice, than for parents to transmit to their children depraved and diseased bodies. Yet how nearly the whole world, the learned and the illiterate alike, high and low, rich and poor, with few exceptions, are wholly thoughtless, improvident, ignorant, and reckless.

As a general rule, this first and most sacred duty of human society is totally disregarded. The great majority of children are the offspring of chance. So far as any intelligent exercise of reason on the part of parents is concerned, they come into the world hap-hazard. They are creatures frequently of lust, rather than love, and very often of mere sensuality in its lowest and most odious sense. And very frequently, too, they are the most unwelcome guests that could be introduced into the family circle.

A child has the right to the inheritance of *absolute health, perfect beauty,* and *complete goodness* of disposition. If it receive not these, it is defrauded of its birthright. And, think you, it will not have its revenge? It certainly will. There is a " law of compensation " pervading all the universe, which harmonizes all apparent discrepancies, which eventually rights all wrongs, which insures in the end penalty to everything done amiss, and reward to every good work, and which secures, ultimately, perfect justice to all. If a parent, through ignorance or viciousness, rob the child of a proper bodily structure, and if society, through heedlessness or selfishness, deprive it of opportunity of normal growth and education, so surely as there is a law in nature and a God in Heaven, it will punish that parent and afflict that society precisely to the extent that it has been wronged. The true physiologist needs but glance at the swarming, vagrant children of our cities, and the frail and puny little ones of the country, to see the operation of this law.

If the people could see this subject in its true light, and if men in authority and in influential positions in society could clearly understand this principle; if ministers of the gospel, whose business it is to point the way to a higher and purer life; if physicians, who claim to be the conservators of the public health; and if teachers, who strive to develop harmoniously all the powers of body and mind, would comprehend this great truth in all of its bearings, our land would not teem with diseased, deformed, ill-born, and ill-bred children, educated to all manner of profligacy, and sure almost to become youthful rowdies and adult vagabonds. But they would see how vastly better and cheaper it would be to train them all to virtue, and educate them to usefulness, than it is to nurture them in evil and then provide them with penitentiaries and prisons.

RESPONSIBILITIES OF PARENTS.

All children would be beautiful if they were healthy, and they would be healthy if their parents were. And all children would be comparatively good also, if, in addition to the health of both parents at the time of conception, the mother was rendered comfortable and happy in all her domestic relations and surrounding circumstances during the period of pregnancy and nursing. A sound mind in a sound body on the part of the parents, and a life of truth and purity, are the conditions which God and nature have appointed.

A married couple should no more allow a child to be conceived when either of them is in a state of fatigue from a hard day's work, or in any condition of bodily exhaustion, or mental disturbance, or agitation, grief, despondency, anxiety, passion, or fretfulness, than they would allow themselves to commit murder. Yet this is done continually; it is rather the rule than the exception in civilized life. And need we wonder at the increasing mortality from still births, marasmus, and convulsions? I have known more than one first child to be born idiotic because of the drinking and feasting which celebrated the wedding occasion.

It is often said by medical writers, and it is the common observation of travelers, that American women are, as a general rule, more frail, more diseased, and more rapidly decaying than the women of any other civilized country on the globe. And this, I fear, is particularly the case with the rising generation of women—the girls. And one of the alarming signs of the times, the increasing disinclination to marry, on the part of the young men of our cities, is very justly attributable to this cause more than to all others.

AMERICAN MOTHERS.

I certainly can intend no flattery to American mothers when I say that, so far as I can learn from reading and observation, there are no mothers on earth who, as a general rule, rear, and govern, and train, and educate, their children so recklessly of all considerations of health, so erroneously in respect to physiological laws, so foolishly in respect to fashion, and so ruinously in respect to consequences, as do American mothers.

This is not, however, *all* their fault. I am not going to put all the blame on her shoulders, nor, indeed, quite half of it. I blame man more for abusing her, and I blame still more the medical profession for misleading both. I regard woman as the victim rather than as the criminal, in relation to the evils I am considering. She has but little opportunity to know any better or do any better than she does. And if, perchance, some woman who has in some way become intelligent on this subject, sets up the standard of truth in her household and dethrones fashion, and attempts to live rationally, and to train up her children healthfully, and objects to give them food or drink which will make them sick, and refuses to have them swallow poisons because they are sick, ten chances to one that friends and neighbors, relatives and doctors, of all the region round about, will come down upon her with an overwhelming avalanche of reproof and ridicule, to say nothing of slang and misrepresentation.

WOMAN'S DISADVANTAGES.

It is not in woman's nature wittingly to sacrifice her child for her own vanity or pleasure ; she will a thousand times sooner sacrifice herself to save her child. Before we condemn her for destroying her own offspring, we must teach her how to save it; and before we blame her for being diseased, we must teach her how, and give her the means, to become healthy.

Man, being more selfish, and taking advantage of the disabilities of woman, consequent on the function of maternity, has monopolized to himself most of the pleasant, wholesome, and profitable vocations, and all of the best educa tional facilities; and thus he is enabled to de velop his intellectual powers; while woman is either made a kitchen drudge or a parlor toy. And when he has reduced her to bodily and mental inferiority, he calls her the " weaker vessel," and says, with stolid self-complacency, " Women are not capable of thinking and reasoning like men."

I blame the medical profession chiefly for woman's disabilities, follies, and infirmities. She has been misled and miseducated by it. She has been taught that she is naturally more frail and feeble and prone to disease than man ; and that she must be dosed and drugged with the most potent poisons for the most trivial indispositions.

THE MEDICAL PROFESSION *vs.* WOMAN.

How does the medical profession treat the efforts of woman to redeem herself from sickness and suffering? A few years ago, a few noble minded women, in view of the dreadful sufferings and great needs of their own sex, and of the confessed inefficiency of the ordinary treatment of the diseases of woman, resolved to qualify themselves, so far as a thorough and *regular* education could do it, for physicians. They were bitterly opposed by the great body of the professors, and most indecently persecuted by the great body of the *gentlemen* medical students. But they persevered; and now schools are established in which women received precisely the same professional education as men, and are graduated according to law. And now the profession is becoming alarmed. They begin to see to what practical result this movement is rapidly tending. It threatens soon to take from it the means whereby it lives. The profession cannot prevent them from getting an education. It cannot control the legislation of the States so as to deprive them of diplomas. There is only one thing it can do; this is to abuse them; and this it seems resolved to do. Will this succeed? Will maltreatment silence her? Will persecution check her? We predict otherwise.

Already a Philadelphia medical society has declared that its members shall not consult with women physicians. A Connecticut medical society has echoed the sentiment. A "reform" medical school has pronounced against the *policy* of educating women to the profession. The Boston *Medical* and *Surgical Journal* opposes woman physicians, and the Edinburgh (Scotland) Medical College has formally voted not to give any diplomas to women.

At the late meeting of the "American Medical Association" in Philadelphia, the physicians of the United States, as represented in that body of self-constituted conservators of the public health, by a majority vote, refused membership to physicians, otherwise unimpeachable, who consulted with doctors of the female sex, or with men of the African race. They even went so far as to ostracize those who taught in medical colleges where women or negroes are educated.

I do not wonder at this opposition; I should wonder if it were not so. Any physician who is sufficiently versed in the technical gibberish of the schools to write a text-book on the "Diseases of Women and Children," or to fill the chair of "Obstetrics and Diseases of Females," can safely prognosticate that, as soon as women get into the profession, a corresponding number of men will get out.

But what objection does her brother make to her as a physician? He raises no question of competency; he does not pretend that she is not quite as successful as himself; he acknowledges that in many respects she has the advantage; he confesses that her constitutional sympathies, her intuitive perceptions, her delicate appreciations, her natural tact and her better opportunities are all in her favor. He does not, and cannot, allege a shadow of a reason why she should not administer to the sufferers of her own sex. And when the women graduates of our school give public lectures, and explain to the people in his presence and in the presence of his patients the fallacies of his doctrines, and the horrid consequences of his treatment, he does not, *and dare not*, gainsay their utterances.

He well knows that the most successful midwives and the most successful practitioners in the diseases peculiar to her sex, in all ages, have been women. But she is accused of being a *woman!* Womanhood is her disqualification!

ORIGIN OF WOMAN'S INFIRMITIES.

Let us look a little into the origin of woman's infirmities, and see precisely what relation there is between the medical profession and her manifold and increasing maladies. And to understand this subject fully, we must trace her history up from the cradle.

During the first four or five years of infancy, the girl baby has nearly the same advantages as the boy baby; but, ever after, the girl is placed at a disadvantage. It is lucky, to begin with, if either girl or boy escapes a serious poisoning at the hands of the doctors before it is a month old. And if any child, in these days of almost constant dosing and drugging, lives a whole year after birth, without being maimed, marred, scarred, stunted, or deformed, by the murderous appliances of the "healing art," such child must be a happy exception to the unfortunate rule. Usually, an infant can not have a cough, a cold, a gripe, a sneeze, or a sniffle, however slight, without the doctor being called. And the doctor does —what? Point out the error in the child's management? ascertain the cause of the trouble and have it removed? instruct the mother or nurse in the laws of Hygiene? Oh! no; nothing of the sort; such *doctoring* would never pay. The profession could not live a year if it gave the mothers of sick babies good advice and withheld bad medicine. And so the doctor does—what? Why, he *poisons the little thing for life!* This is what is expected of him; it is what he is employed to do, and he does it. And here is "original sin" in the physiological, or, rather, the pathological sense. Here is the "origin of evil" in the vital domain; the first great act of disobedience which is sure, sooner or later, to bring death and many woes into the family circle.

Several thousands of young drug doctors are

turned out from the medical colleges annually to do—what? To teach the world how to avoid disease? to be the exemplars of the laws of life? to educate the people in the conditions of health? to instruct the people how to avoid the causes of disease? to preach obedience to the laws of nature? Not at all. They are as ignorant of these things as the people are. They are themselves among the chief transgressors; their precepts and their examples are only leading the world more rapidly to perdition. Grim Death has no more efficient emissaries. They go forth "poisoning and to poison." If a baby is sick, they poison it; if it continues sick, they poison it again. If the sickness is prolonged, they multiply these poisons; and when the drug diseases supersede or supervene upon the original disease, the doctors have an unlimited field of practice before them in drugging the symptoms of the drug diseases.

One common-sensical mother or unsophisticated nurse is worth more than a regiment of young drug doctors, or old ones either, for sick babies. If any unusual pestilence—cholera, plague, or diptheria—should send to premature graves during the ensuing year, one half as many children as the doctors kill with their drug-poisons, a panic which would bring people to their prayers if not to their reason would pervade all the land.

When the boy and girl arrive at the age of seven, eight, or ten years, the disadvantages of a fashionable education which regards fashion and "accomplishments" as superior to health and utility, become conspicuous. The boy is provided with mechanical tools; he is taken into the fields and woods, and made acquainted with animals and machinery, farms and workshops. He runs, jumps, climbs trees, rides horses, drives oxen, works, plays, and develops his muscles while he expands his mind in a thousand ways. Thus he observes, compares, analyzes, reflects, and treasures up useful knowledge; and thus he learns to work his way, to accomplish his purposes, to overcome obstacles, to subdue opposition, to achieve success, to develop himself.

But the little girl, what of her? She is shut up in the nursery, or seated quietly in the parlor with a doll-baby to study, and, perchance, a kitten for a companion. If she is irritable, and peevish, and sick, as she cannot help being, she is fed on candy and lozenges, and stuffed with sweet-cake. She is taught that little girls should dress up, sit still, and be pretty. She is told that it is vulgar to run and jump; that only little boys are fitted to do out-door work or enjoy out-door play; and thus she is deprived of the only possible means of acquiring a good constitution, and of giving to the mental powers a high and ennobling direction. And yet she is expected to be the mother of the race. She may be the mother of a race.

She is to a great extent blasted, dwarfed, and perverted, in childhood; and just to that extent must her womanhood, if ever attained, be imperfect. She is made to believe that young gentlemen are expected to act usefully, think rationally, feel normally, and do business; and that young ladies are made to be accomplished, feel amiable, follow the fashions, and get—*married*. Too often, before she is sufficiently developed for a husband she gets the *consumption*. And when, as the result of her miseducation, her intellect becomes disordered, her feelings morbid, her judgment unreliable, her disposition eccentric, and her fancies fantastic, she is complacently told by those who have made her what she is—

"Frailty, thy name is woman."

DRESS AND RESPIRATION.

As the girl grows up to womanhood, she is hampered and trammeled with a style of dress which renders it utterly impossible for her to exercise properly or breathe freely. Heavy skirts drag down and displace the abdominal and pelvic viscera, and a "decent fit" around the waist prevents the normal play of the respiratory organs.

Says A. K. Gardiner, M. D., of New York: "So soon as the sex of the child is made evident by any external manipulations of dress, so soon does the bodily degeneracy commence. Look at the dress of woman! Were man so to direct the fashion of woman's dress in order to enable him, by physical force, to overcome her and tyrannize over her, he could not more completely fetter her than she shackles herself."

You may measure any woman's available power by her breathing capacity, and her digestive power is precisely proportioned to her respiration; and the circulation and purity of blood is dependent on respiration, and nutrition is governed by the circulation; and thus the very structures of the body are dependent on the amount of air taken into the lungs.

As a general rule, the men of America are vastly better developed in the breathing apparatus than are the women; and this disproportion is greater with the people of the United States than with the people of any other nation on the globe. Contrast the full, rounded busts, the plump arms and rosy cheeks of the majority of Irish and German, and even English women in this country, with the narrow, tapering waists and "caved-in" vital organs of native American women—I do not mean *Indians*, for I have yet to see the first specimen of a narrow chest in a red woman.

It is of vastly more importance to society and to the race that woman should be well developed in the respiratory organs than it is that man should be; she has to breathe for more than herself.

While in the embryo state, the child must receive its oxygen from the air which the mother
inspires.   Many a strong, vigorous mother has
given birth to a frail, scrofulous child, because
she was so plethoric, or sedentary, that she only
breathed enough for herself.   If either parent is
to be restrained in the vital region and deprived
of the breath of life, let it not be the one who is
to nourish from her own blood and impress her
own organic conditions on the future generations.

The history of Miss Harriet Hosmer, the eminent sculptress, is instructive here.   Her father,
an eminent physician of Watertown, Mass., had
lost wife and children of consumption, and fear-
ing a like fate for Harriet, who was now the only
survivor, he gave her dog, gun, and boat, and in-
sisted on an out-door life as indispensable to
health.   She willingly acquiesced in her father's
plans, and pursued her sports so energetically
that she soon became a fearless horsewoman, a
good shot, and an adept in rowing, swimming,
diving, and skating.   She had also other inducements to open-air exercise, for, "many a time
and oft, she might have been found in a certain
clay-pit, not far from the parental residence, making early attempts at modeling horses, dogs, sheep,
men and women, or any object which attracted
her attention."

Had Miss Hosmer been subjected to the ordinary treatment of girls or been doctored in the usu-

al method for consumptives, she would, in all prob-
ability, have perished in early life ; but, " under
the regimen which her father so wisely devised
for her, she gradually acquired health and strength,
and has reached the years of mature womanhood
with a well-developed and robust body, and with
a mind full of earnest purpose, noble ambition,
and the most untiring energy and perseverance."

If we could induce all of the fathers and mothers of our country to dismiss all of their drug-
doctors, and to give their children a physiological
education, those ever-present and still increasing
pestilences, scrofula and consumption, would
nearly disappear in the next generation, and entirely, in another.

DRESS AND THE SEXUAL FUNCTIONS.

As self-preservation is the first law of nature,
those parents who damage their own constitutions and waste their vital stamina by unhygienic
habits, dissipation or poisonous drugs, deprive
their offspring of a proper organization. Many
persons, perhaps a majority, seem to suppose that
it makes little difference with offspring what
they do to themselves—that individual life and
health have little or nothing to do with the reproductive function. But it has everything to do
with it. Individual life must first be provided
for, and if vitality is exhausted, or vitalizing

rèsources deficient, it is the offspring that suffers most.

The disastrous effects of fashionable dress on the sexual organs and functions directly, and on the integrity and welfare of the race indirectly, is a subject on which physiologists have but one opinion, and on which medical men of all schools agree.

I quote the following words of fearful import, from the latest standard work on the diseases of women; a work just published by Henry A. Lea, of Philadelphia. The author is Professor T. Gaillard Thomas, M. D., of New York. Dr. Thomas says (page 58) : "The dress adopted by the women of our times may be very graceful and becoming, it may possess the great advantages of developing the beauties of the figure and concealing its defects, but it certainly is conducive to the development of uterine diseases, and proves not merely a predisposing but an exciting cause of them. For the proper performance of the function of respiration, an entire freedom of action should be given to the chest, and more especially is this needed at the base of the thorax, opposite the attachment of the important respiratory muscle, the diaphragm. The habit of contracting the body at the waist by tight clothing confines this part as if by splints; indeed, it accomplishes just what the surgeon does who bandages the chest for a fractured rib, with the intent of limiting thoracic and substituting abdominal respiration.

"As the diaphragm, thus fettered, contracts, all lateral expansion being prevented, it presses the intestines upon the movable uterus, and forces this organ down upon the floor of the pelvis, or lays it across it. In addition to the force thus exerted, a number of pounds, say from five to ten, are bound around the contracted waist, and held up by the hips and the abdominal walls, which are rendered protuberant by the compression alluded to. The uterus is exposed to this downward pressure for fourteen hours out of every twenty-four; at stated intervals being still further pressed upon by a distended stomach.

"In estimating the effects of direct pressure upon the position of the uterus, its extreme mobility must be constantly borne in mind. No more striking evidence of this can be cited than the fact, that in examining it by Sim's speculum, the cervix is thrown so far back into the bottom of the sacrum as to make its engagement in the field of the instrument often very difficult, and that attention to this point in the arrangement of the patient will at once remove the difficulty. While the uterus is exposed by the speculum, it will be found to ascend with every expiratory effort, and descend with every inspiration; and so distinct and constant are the rapid alterations of position thus induced, that in operations in the vaginal canal the surgeon can tell with great certainty how respiration is being affected by the anæsthetic employed. An organ so easily and decidedly influenced as to position by such slight causes must necessarily be affected by a constriction which, in autopsy, will sometimes be found to have left the impress of the ribs upon the liver, producing depressions corresponding to them.

" No one will charge me with drawing upon my imagination, even in the remotest degree, for the details of the following picture; for a little reflection will assure all of its correctness. A lady, who has habitually dressed as already described, prepares for a ball by increasing all the evil influences which result from pressure. Although she may be menstruating, she dances until a late hour of the night, or rather an early hour of the morning. She then eats a hearty supper, passes out into the inclement night air, and rides a long distance to her home. This is repeated frequently during each season, until advancing age or the occurrence of disease puts an end to the process.

" A great deal of exposure is likewise entailed upon women by the uncovered state of the lower extremities. The body is covered, but under the skirts sweeps a chilling blast, and from the wet earth rises a moist vapor that comes in contact with limbs encased in thin cotton cloth, which is entirely inadequate for protection. It is not surprising that evil often results to a menstruating woman thus constantly exposed."

SHOULD FASHIONABLE WOMEN MARRY?

The work of Dr. Thomas is intended as a text-book for physicians. But the following words, delicate or indelicate, ought to be read by every young person in the land who contemplates matrimony:

" To a woman who has systematically displaced her uterus by years of imprudence, the act of sexual intercourse, which, in one whose organs maintain a normal position, is a physiological process devoid of pathological results, *becomes an absolute and positive source of disease*. The axis of the uterus is not identical with that of the vagina. While the latter has an axis co-incident with that of the inferior strait, the former has one similar to the superior. This arrangement provides for the passage of the male organ below the cervix into the posterior cul-de-sac, the cervix thus escaping injury. But let the uterus be forced down, as it is by the prevailing styles of fashionable dress, even to the distance of one inch, and the natural state of the parts is altered. The cervix is directly injured, and thus a physiological process is insensibly merged into one productive of pathological results. How often do we see uterine disease occur just after matrimony, even where no excesses have been committed. It is not an excessive indulgence in coition which so often produces this result, but the indulgence *to any degree* on the part of a woman who has disturbed the natural relations of the genital organs."

All that Dr. Thomas affirms or implies is fully corroborated by other authors. In a work on Woman and her Diseases, by the late Professor Charles D. Meigs, of Jefferson Medical College, Philadelphia, the author makes the remark that, the pressure resulting from prolapsus of the uterus for half an inch often produces intolerable agony.

DRUGGING AT PUBERTY.

If the girl survive her infantile drugging, her mal-training and her miseducation, and grows up to womanhood, the disadvantages of false fashions and the evils of a false medical system follow. She is imperiled at every step. At the period of puberty an important change occurs in the development of the organism; she becomes fitted for another range of functional processes, and is at this time liable to periodical indisposition. These ailments—difficulties in menstruation—are usually trifling, and are caused mainly by sedentary habits, dietetic errors, especially constipating food, overexertion, colds, &c. A little proper attention to diet, exercise, ventilation, bathing, &c., would, in almost all cases, remove them in a short time.

But, instead of this, the doctor is called upon, and emmenagogues, or "forcing medicines," are resorted to. The patient is sorely and sadly damaged with the preparations of iron, mercury, iodine, antimony, and opium, or other narcotics, when a warm bath or a fomentation, with rest and quiet for a day or two, were all that nature required. And here is the origin of many distressing chronic diseases of the reproductive organs, which often render the patient infirm and miserable for life. The extensive and in creasing prevalence of uterine diseases and displacements is attributable to the drugs adminis tered for the trivial ailments which attend the early stages of the menstrual effort, more than to all other causes combined, with the exception of fashionable dress. I have had scores of bedridden women to treat, whose long years of chronic disease, uterine inflammation and ulceration, prolapsus and other displacements, utter helplessness and dreary future, were all and wholly owing to a few weeks' drugging at fifteen or sixteen years of age.

I have never found any difficulty in speedily overcoming all the disorders of incipient menstruation by means of hygienic appliances, when all drugs were kept out of the way.

SCIENTIFIC DRUGGERY.

People are little aware of the horrible mischief which is produced by the ordinary *scientific* treatment of the diseases of woman. A brief glance at the authorities may shed more light on the terrible delusion which prevails here than a long argument; all can understand facts, though few may appreciate logic. Let us see precisely what are the *remedies* which are recommended by the standard authors, and approved by the text-books of medical schools.

One of the late standard authorities is " The Disease of Females, by Fleetwood Churchill, M. D., F. R. S.," and it reflects very fully and very fairly the prevailing practice of the profession. It should be remarked that all of the maladies under consideration are conditions of weakness and obstruction—so recognized by all authors. By whatever name the disorder may be known in the nosological arrangement, or by whatever cause it may have been produced, its essential elements are obstruction, or debility, or both. Well, then, what shall the medical man do to remove obstructions and invigorate the functions? Churchill recommends for—

Amenorrhœa.—Bleeding, leeches, cupping, blisters, aloes, assafetida, wine, iodine, ergot, carbonate of iron, copperas, metallic iron, madder, strychnine, cantharides, turpentine, savin, aconite.

Vicarious Menstruation.—Leeches, cupping, blisters, muriatic acid, aqua fortis, oil of vitriol, aloes, iron, opium, sugar of lead.

Dysmenorrhœa.—Bleeding, leeches, cupping, blisters, caustics, opium, scarifications, morphine, henbane, poison hemlock, camphor, Indian hemp, acetate of ammonia, ergot, alcohol, preparations of iron, zinc, tincture of Spanish flies, borax, hellebore, senega, snake root, salts, mercury, iodine, tartar emetic.

Menorrhagia.—Bleeding, leeches, cupping, opium, sugar of lead, ergot, Indian hemp, ipecac, blue pill, elixir vitriol, sulphuric acid, nitric acid, hydrochloric acid, iron, copperas, logwood, drastic purgatives, gallic acid, oxide of silver, nettle juice, turpentine.

Cessation of Menstruation.—Leeches, blisters, issues, setons, purgatives, hydrochlorate of ammonia.

Chlorosis.—Blisters, mercurial inunction, rhubarb, aloetic purgatives, ammonia, metallic iron, copperas, iodide of iron, chalybeate spring water, tannate of iron, citrate of iron, lactate of iron, proto-muriate of iron, hydrochlorate of iron, blue pill, henbane, mineral tonics generally, vegetable tonics generally, glauber salts.

Leucorrhœa.—Leeches, cupping, blisters, balsam, copaiba, copperas, muriate of iron, ergot, logwood, cubebs, colchicum, crab's eyes, Spanish flies, conium, iodine, opium, henbane, lunar caustic.

Irritable Uterus.—Leeches, cupping, blisters, scarifications, henbane, deadly nightshade, camphor, assafetida, mercury, arsenic.

All of these prescriptions amount to nothing more nor less than an indiscriminate routine of the most deadly drugs and destructives to be found in the *materia medica.* But the great question back of all this is, Do these things cure? We have the testimony at hand which settles this question in the negative.

SCANZONI *vs.* CHURCHILL.

There has recently been issued from the press an elaborate work—a work of nearly seven hundred pages, on "The Diseases of the Sexual Organs of Woman," by F. W. Von Scanzoni, Professor of Midwifery and Diseases of Females in the University of Wurzburg, Counselor to His Majesty the King of Bavaria, Chevalier of many Orders, translated from the French of Drs. H. Dorr and A. Socin, and annoted with the approval of the author, by Augustus R. Gardner, A. M., M. D., Professor of Clinical Midwifery and the Diseases of Woman, in the New York Medical College, author of "The Causes and Curative Treatment of Sterility;" editor of "Tyler Smith's Lectures on Obstetrics;" etc.

The work of Dr. Scanzoni is the largest and the latest European work which the medical profession has given to the world on the diseases

of woman; and the imposing parade of author-
ship ought to satisfy the most incredulous that
the statements of the author are entitled to re-
spectful consideration.

Well, what does the learned professor, who has
had so large an experience in the treatment of
the diseases we have named, say of the ordinary
remedies ? I extract his testimony in relation to
a single one of these ailments, *Hysteralgia*. It
is in the following words :—

"We have almost exhausted all the series of
medicaments recommended in the books of mod
ern authors; narcotics in large doses; powerful
purgatives, iron, mercurials, quinine, arsenic, and
many other means we have tried *without the
least result*. Topical applications have been no
more useful. We have omitted neither deep
scarifications of the mouth of the womb, so much
recommended, nor the applications of leeches, nor
the dilatation of the cervical canal, by means of
sounds and prepared sponge; the introduction of
narcotic agents or pieces of ice into the vagina;
lavements of the tincture of opium and the extract of belladonna, etc., etc., *but all without relief.* Only *once* we produced *some* relief to a
patient by the local application of the fumes of
chloroform; but this good effect *was not of long
duration.*"

Could any commentary add force to this sting-
ing condemnation of the popular practice ?

Well might Dr. Ramage, of the London Royal College, pronounce the whole system of drug-medication a "burning shame to its professors."

We must, however, in candor, acknowledge that, within a few years, the evidence of drug-medication has been somewhat investigated, especially with American physicians, and that the later authors recommend drug poisons in less variety and diminished quantity. But whether this improvement has resulted from the progress of Homeopathy, the diffusion of hygienic intelligence, the disinclination on the part of the patient to swallow the drugs, or the observation of their disastrous consequences on the part of the drug doctors, or of all of these influences combined, we need not speculate. Humanity's hope is that this step in the right direction will be succeeded by other similar ones until the blessed ultimatum of NO DRUGGERY is reached.

But, on referring to the treatment of menstrual diseases, as explained in the recent able work of Dr. Thomas, we see there is still room enough for improvement, as the frightful list of toxicological agents which he recommends will show. They are as follows :—

For Dysmenorrhœa.—Colchicum, guaiac, bleeding, preparations of iron, Indian hemp, hydrate of chloral, belladonna, assafetida, opium, mercury, iodine, nitrate of silver, carbolic acid.

For Menorrhagia.—Elixir vitriol, opium, sulphuric acid, gallic acid, ergot, Indian hemp, preparations of iron, alum, tannin, mercury, bleeding, iodine, nitric acid, muriatic acid.

Amenorrhœa.—Bleeding, preparations of iron, strychnia, quinine, aloes, myrrh, rue, savin, ergot.

Leucorrhœa.—Bleeding, persulphate of iron, alum, tannin, oak bark, zinc, lead.

Chlorosis.—Arsenic, strychnine, quinine, saccharated carbonate of iron, iron by hydrogen, bitter wine of iron, potassa, wine, whisky, malt liquors.

It is a "poor pathology, and worse practice," that can unite the standard medical authorities of the world in prescribing *arsenic, mercury, strychnine, iron,* and bleeding, for nearly all the ills that woman's flesh is heir to. Was there not as much truth as poetry in the declaration of Professor Oliver Wendell Holmes, M. D., which so astounded and confounded the Massachusetts Medical Society that "mankind have been literally drugged to death"?

DR. PRESCOTT ON DRUGGERY.

After a lecture to ladies, in Boston, in March, 1862, I called on the venerable Dr. Prescott of Farmington, Me., who happened to be present, to state the conclusions of his experience. He readily responded, and stated that in reviewing the results of an extensive practice in all forms of diseases of women, he could not ascertain that a single case of many thousands had ever been cured or materially benefited by drug medication, either in his own practice or in that of his professional brethren. On the contrary, multitudes had been sadly damaged, and many killed outright. Dr. Prescott is known throughout New England as a physician of large experience, and as a man of irreproachable integrity. Twelve years previously he repudiated druggery, and has since practiced the hygienic system.

DRUGGING IN ACUTE DISEASES.

But in chronic diseases, in which the patient may be dragged toward death for five, ten, or twenty years, and "still live," the fatal tendency of the practice cannot be very well understood by the non-professional people. They are very apt to think, and generally do think, that the very medicines which have produced all of their maladies, after the first one, and ruined their constitutions, have really saved their lives a dozen of times. And the more they are damaged and diseased by the drug-poisons, the louder the deluded victims clamor for more.

Let us see, then, how drug medication works in acute diseases, where death or recovery must be determined in a few days; and for an illustration, I select the disease called *puerperal fever.* There is much discrepancy in the profession respecting the "seat" and *pathology*—as it is called

—of this disease; but all are agreed that it is essentially an acute inflammation of some portion of the abdominal or pelvic viscera or structures, with an accompanying fever. But this concord in nosology does not lessen the discord in therapy, for two exactly opposite methods of treatment are recommended by the highest medical authorities. Professor Alonzo Clark, M. D., of the New York College of Physicians and Surgeons, earnestly advises active stimulation, while Professor Charles D. Meigs, M. D., of the Jefferson Medical College of Philadelphia, as strenuously insists on copious depletion. The stimulating plan consists of opium, brandy, quinine, calomel, etc., internally; and hot flannel, turpentine, etc., externally. The depleting plan consists of bleeding, salts, veratrum, digitalis, etc.

Now, if one of these methods of treatment is right, the other is certainly wrong. But the exact truth is, they are both wrong. The patient has a much better chance to live under no treatment than under either plan. And the fatality attending the disease—more than one-half the cases terminating in death—is, at least, presumptive evidence against both kinds of medication.

PROFESSOR GILMAN ON PUERPERAL FEVER.

And here the testimony and experience of Professor Gilman, of the New York College of Physicians and Surgeons, are valuable and significant.

In a classical lecture to his medical class, in the winter of 1862, Dr. Gilman said :—

" Mild cases will recover under any treatment ; severe cases die under all treatment. You are therefore justified in trying any plan you can think of. In Bellevue Hospital, twenty-two out of twenty-three patients have died. In the Paris and London hospitals, seventy-five per cent die. One physician had ninety-five cases, and *lost them all.*"

This statement concerning the mortality of this disease, so far as the Parisian hospitals are concerned, is corroborated by Anna Inman, M. D., a graduate of the Hygeio-Therapeutic College, who spent a year in the hospitals of that city.

Professor Simpson, of Edinburgh, Scotland, states, in *Braithwaite's Retrospect* for January, 1861, that three thousand mothers die annually in England and Wales, during the lying-in period, and a majority of them of *puerperal fever.*

With regard to the treatment of the disease, Dr. Gilman recommends opium, not because he has any faith in it, or in anything else, but because he can administer it with "less of the *blackness of despair.*" He recommends, also, hot poultices, but objects to bleeding. He regards turpentine as exceedingly pernicious and distressing. He would rather keep the patient under chloroform. He condemns calomel. He says that veratrum will reduce the pulse from 140 to

100, but in a few hours the *patient is dead*. Such facts and figures require no comment. If the reader cannot understand the lesson taught in their naked presentation, he would not believe though ten thousand should rise from their graves, and declare themselves to have been the victims of

"The deadly virtues of the healing art."

DRUGGING DURING PREGNANCY.

But if the woman escapes with dear life the ailments incident to puberty, other perils are before her. In the common order of events, the matrimonial relation is formed. Then come child-birth and nursing, with all their joys and sorrows. Lucky is the woman who can, on these occasions, escape the doctor's lancet and drugs. During pregnancy, she usually suffers more or less of nausea, cramps, constipation, vertigo, etc., for which she is bled, physicked, and narcotized, predisposing her to hemorrhage, milk-leg, broken breast, and other *sequelæ*, and multiplying the occasions for taking more medicines.

DRUGGING DURING THE LYING-IN PERIOD.

After confinement, the majority of women are troubled (and no wonder) more or less with indigestion, constipation, sour stomach, flatulence, sore mouth, sick headache, etc., for which chalk, soda, saleratus, magnesia, lunar caustic, bismuth, blue pill, etc., are prescribed. And now the medicines are doing a double work of mischief. These drugs which she is continually taking into her system, under the name of medicine, deprave the blood, vitiate all of the secretions, and poison the very fountain whence the new-born being derives its nourishment.

. These drug poisons must be expelled. The living system gets rid of them through every available channel. And that portion which passes off with the milk often destroys the life of the nursing infant, or renders it a puny, feeble thing for life.

So much for the child. It must be at all times liable to canker, colic, humors, rashes, convulsions, and death, so long as its mother is continually taking into her system that which contaminates and impoverishes the only source of its subsistence.

CHRONIC DRUG DISEASE.

But if the mother survives the terrible ordeal which a false medical system imposes on her, there is yet trouble enough in the future. The dosings of infancy, the druggings of puberty, and the poisonings of her maternity, have laid the foundations for innumerable and nameless chronic diseases ; and now these must be doctored *secundum artem.* And thus medical science has laid the foundation for an extensive practice in the healing art—provided the patient lives long enough.

In due time, the woman comes to be regarded as a *confirmed invalid.* And no sooner is she " cured " of one malady, than another " sets in."

How strange that some new disease is always ready to " supervene " so soon as the existing one is " subdued !" Her aches and pains, and " sinking spells," and flutterings, and *gonenesses,* and short breathings, and palpitations, and dragging sensations, and nervousness, require, in the judgment of the family physician, a course of tonics, nervines, and stimulants, and quassia, carbonate of ammonia, assafetida, castor, musk, valerian, spices, aromatics, phosphate of iron, or iron-by-hydrogen, wine, brandy, porter, ale, lager beer, etc., etc.

She is also put on the medico-slop diet of the pharmacopœias—fed on such delicate abominations as panada, starch puddings, beef tea, mutton broth, oyster soup, chicken gravy, buttered toast, and sugar nick-nacks. In a word, instead of being nourished and strengthened, she is merely stuffed and stimulated.

All this makes a bad matter worse ; and at length the doctor, having treated the *general dyspeptic condition* for a few months, or a few years, looks a little deeper into the case, and finds out that the patient has a *torpid liver.* Then come

calomel and opium, perhaps blue pill again, to
" touch up " the hepatic function, with henbane,
or conium, or morphia, to quiet the irritation.

Well, in due time the torpid liver is " cured,"
or its action so depressed that it ceases to make
any further resistance to the medicines, and now
the doctor discovers that *jaundice* has " set in."
Verily it has. And the drugs are just what have
set it in. But this jaundice must be " treated;"
and so the persevering physician doses it, or the
patient, with a combination of " alteratives "—
antimony, hydriodate of potassa, yellow dock,
bitter sweet, blue flag, mandrake, black cohosh,
corrosive sublimate, iodine, and arsenic.

And thus another set of poisons are sent into
the vital domain, with the inevitable result of
another set of drug diseases. Soon, another
diagnosis is made, and the disease is pronounced
kidney complaint. This is medicated with
leeches, cuppings, salts, antiphlogistics, diuretics,
alkalies and counter irritants, and the next phase
of the malady is said to be *nervous debility.*
And again the patient must be put on tonics,
stimulants, and nervines, as lunar caustic, phos-
phorus, ammonia, extract of hops, cascarilla,
myrrh, hypophosphites, preparations of iron, camphor, ether, spirits of nitre, compound spirits of
lavender, golden seal, unicorn, wormwood, thor-
oughwort, skunk cabbage, etc., etc.

When the sensibility of the nervous system is

sufficiently subdued, the nervous debility is as *subdued* also. The disease is " cured," though the patient is nearly killed ; but no sooner is the cure achieved than (how unfortunate !) still another disease " supervenes." Now the muscular system gives out; the back becomes weak, and the limbs tremulous. The kind and ever-faithful physician now diagnosticates *spinal irritation*. Still he is not without hope for his patient. The resources of his art are immense. There are in the apothecary shop at least one thousand drugs which he has not yet administered, and there are numerous processes which he has not yet brought into requisition. Why should he be discouraged ? So long as there is life there is hope—at least of making a bill.

Blistering, cupping, leeching, scarifying, pustulations, caustics, issues, setons moxa burnings and the actual cautery, are the *scientific* remedies for spinal irritation.

The marring, and scarring, and haggling, and mangling, finally *overcome* the spinal irritation, and then we come to the end of the chapter, which is *neuralgia*.

Neuralgia is regarded as incurable. But there is one consolation—there are no more diseases to "set in." The patient has got below the range of their action, and hence can not be " attacked " by them. Her vitality is too low to respond to morbific causes, hence they may remain in her system without any special effort to get rid of them. She cannot, therefore, have any particular disease known to the nosology, but she can be very wretched.

The doctors can cure almost everything except neuralgia. We have seen how effectually they cure dyspepsia, liver complaint, jaundice, kidney disease, nervous debility and spinal irritation, but neuralgia is peculiarly a "medicorum opprobrium." Yet medical science does not wholly despair, it can still "alleviate the symptoms." For what did "nature provide" morphine, quinine, stramonium, belladonna, prussic acid, veratria, aconite, chloroform, digitalis, henbane, ratsbane, dogsbane, fleabane, and all the banes, venoms and viruses, all the drugs and die stuffs, and dregs and scum of the mineral, vegetable, and animal kingdoms, except to quiet pain? And so long as the poor patient is dosed with narcotics and depressants below the point of susceptibility, she may be kept oblivious of misery. Has not medicine been entitled *the art divine?* I fear the Irish doctor was not far wrong when he presented a bill to his wealthy neighbor: "To curing your wife till she died."

And now after medical skill has done its best, or its worst, surgical ingenuity exhausts itself in vam efforts to repair the damages occasioned by bad living and worse doctoring. The uterine organs become permanently congested, relaxed, and debilitated, ulcerations occur, excrescences form, and displacements result.

These are treated indiscriminately with astringents, caustics, pessaries, braces, leechings, scarifyings and burnings, which, although in some cases temporary relief is obtained, never fail to aggravate the difficulties in the end.

Induration paralysis, fistulous openings, extensive inflammations, permanent adhesions, fungous excrescences, and cancerous ulcerations, are among the frightful catalogue of evils which result from these attempts to give " mechanical support " to the displaced viscera.

Not long since, I had a patient under treatment for erosive or cancerous degeneration of the uterus, the consequence of the prolonged employment of pessaries. And a few years ago, I was consulted by a lady who had a fistulous ulcer opening externally from the bowels, just below the umbilicus, through which the fecal matters were discharged, produced by wearing an " abdominal supporter."

A few years ago, I visited a young lady in Philadelphia who had been a bed-ridden invalid for fifteen years, in consequence of a retroversion of the womb. Her father was wealthy, and had employed the most eminent physicans and surgeons of that doctor-making city, who had invented a bureau drawer full of "supporters" for the displaced organ; and they had "toned her

up" with tonics, and "quieted her down" with
nervines, and nourished her on "blood food"
preparations of iron, until her muscular system
was as limsy as a wet rag. And these are but
examples of hundreds whose cases have come
under my observation and treatment.

I cannot pursue this branch of my subject here.
Those who would have fuller information are re-
ferred to my larger works, "Pathology of the
Reproductive Organs," and "Uterine Diseases
and Displacements." The limits of this work
will only enable me to show the errors and ab-
surdities of the prevailing medical system and
indicate

THE BETTER WAY.

If I should succeed in inducing all who are afflicted with the maladies under consideration to
abandon drug-medication of every kind, at once
and forever, leaving them in all other respects to
the same influences, I should be the means of
saving many lives and an incalculable amount of
suffering; but I propose to do more. Almost all
of these ailments are readily curable by hygienic
appliances. The exceptions are very few, and
confined almost wholly to the cases in which the
patients' vitality has been nearly all drugged out
of them. Indeed, I seldom find any serious difficulty in managing the cases, so far as the original maladies are concerned; but it not unfre-

quently happens that the drug-poisons have made such ravages on the constitutional stamina, that the patient, although capable of being rendered comfortable, can never be made vigorous. These patients often come to us with only the *remains* of a shattered organism, and seem to expect that we can, by some marvelous, if not miraculous, "cold-water" process, reconstruct them as good as new.

But this can not be done. Vitality once lost can never be regained. Says Professor Clarke, of the New York College of Physicians and surgeons: "All of our medicines are poisons, and as a consequence every dose diminishes the patient's vitality." Let those who have suffered a diminution of vitality one hundred or one thousand times in this way, calculate, if they can, the aggregate loss, and then let them reflect on the declaration of Professor Draper, of the New York University Medical School: "Vitality once lost can never be regained."

All that our system can do for the abused organism of these miserable sufferers is to put them in healthy conditions. We can restore them to the normal use of all there is left of themselves; and this is much. It is often the transition, as it were, from death unto life; from wretchedness unto happiness.

When I am asked what I would do or have done to a woman suffering any form of disease peculiar to her sex, I invariably answer, First of all, *stop taking medicine.* Cease to do evil. There is not one woman in a thousand, provided she is not already death-struck, who has been in the habit of taking medicine for years, who will not improve at once on discontinuing it entirely. Many hundreds have told me the same story, and I have yet to find the first exception; and there are few adult persons who can not refer to such cases within the circle of their acquaintance.

Sometimes patients who have been drug-doctored five or ten years, leave off medicine in very despair; in other cases, their physicians become absolutely tired of drugging them, and abandon them to their fate; but I never knew nor heard of such a discontinuance of druggery that was not followed by an immediate improvement of the patient's health.

But the patient need not be limited to this merely negative advantage; she may perchance adopt the appliances of the True Healing Art, remedial even beyond her most sanguine expectations. The letters I have received from wives and mothers, who had endured half a life of disease, doctors' drugs, and misery, but who are now in the enjoyment of health, happiness, and happy homes, could be counted by thousands.

Nor is the Hygienic treatment so afflicting a dispensation as many have been led to believe. The majority of patients at a good establishment are more comfortable under treatment than they could be without. It is the only place where some of them can be out of misery. The whole discipline of a properly conducted institution and the whole management of the patient are calculated to render her sensations more agreeable, and life more enjoyable. It is very true that, in the first instance, some patients suffer for a short time the deprivation of accustomed stimuli; but this is soon and amply compensated by the restoration of the normal sensations, giving a keen relish for the simplest aliments. She must abandon tea, coffee, grease and gravies, candies and confections, all forms of constipating food and all stimulating beverages. The stomach must be no longer a drug-shop, nor a common reservoir for all the unclean things and indigestible trash of the shops and market places.

Those things which have normal relations to the living system should be employed as remedial agents, instead of those materials which are incompatible with vital organs. Unleavened bread must take the place of aloes and rhubarb; good fruit must be taken instead of jalap and cream of tartar; fresh air must supersede squills and ipecac; exercise must substitute gum drops and lager-beer; sleep must be resorted to instead of morphine; pure, soft water must expel salts and antimony; bathing and friction be employed in

lieu of liniment and rubefacients, and paralyzing
machinery be exchanged for vitalizing manipulations.   Temperance in all things must stop the
waste of vital power, and obedience to organic
law arrest the premature decay of the organic
tissues.

TOBACCO *vs.* WOMAN.

I cannot conclude this subject without advert-
ing very briefly to another evil whose disastrous
effects on the health of many women seem to be
very little understood.   I mean *tobacco-using by
men.*   I know that I am liable here of being
suspected of an attempt at exaggeration—at
straining a point—but I undertake to say that
thousands of women and children are rendered
miserable invalids, and that some are killed outright, by the poisonous breath and pestilent perspiration of tobacco-smoking-and-chewing husbands and fathers.

Those who do not use tobacco are vastly more
sensitive to its influence than those who do.
They cannot come in contact with its deleterious
fumes without being more or less irritated; and
the purer their instincts, and the less gross their
habits of living, the more acutely will they feel
its injurious influence.

You know how it is with the experienced liquor drinker; he can often swallow a pint of
brandy, or a quart of whisky, or a keg of lager.

a day, and still keep about, and imagine himself sober, and not be aware of any foulness of stomach or lungs, of blood or brains; yet the horrid stench of his breath may disgust and sicken one who is not addicted to the habit.

The veteran tobacco sot has so stupefied his senses, and perverted his instincts, that he can hold a quid of the filthy weed in both corners of his mouth, and a pipe or cigar between them, and find the sensations the most delightful that his gross nature is capable of realizing, when to all uncontaminated noses he is as offensive as a cesspool. Every breath of air that a tobacco-smoking man exhales from his lungs, and every particle of perspiration that a tobacco-chewing man emits from his skin, is loaded with deadly poison. And here is the rationale of many nervous, irritable, and declining women. They seldom know, their husbands rarely suspect, and their drug doctors never imagine, what causes the trouble.

I have had many patients who had become dyspeptic, hysterical, afflicted frequently with vertigo, syncope, and various "strange spells" which I could and did readily trace to the virulent emanations of their tobacco-using "bosom companions." On putting the twain asunder for a few weeks, and subjecting the "better halves" to the proper processes of purification, they would rapidly recover health, and soon be ready to return to their loving lords to be poisoned again in the same way. I have been obliged to offend some husbands by declaring to them that they must either get a divorce from their tobacco, occupy apartments separate from their wives, or see their wives die in a year or two of consump tion.

One of the most deplorable signs of the times is the rapidly increasing prevalence of this most detestable and disgusting vice among the young men of our country. And if the American women, maids and matrons, do not soon exert themselves to persuade or shame their lovers, husbands, and sons, out of the habit of tobacco-using, the nation, if not the race, is as surely doomed as there is a law in nature or a God in the universe.

Yet if fathers smoke and chew tobacco, why should not their sons? And if fathers and sons, why not mothers and daughters? If the old use it, why not the young? If doctors and ministers smoke tobacco, why should not their patients and their flocks imitate their example? If the leaders and teachers of the people smoke, why should not the people themselves smoke, and society go to perdition in one universal tobacco smudge?

GLOSSARY.

Abdominal. Pertaining to the bowels.

Aconite. Wolf's bane ; a poisonous plant.

Alterative. That which restores healthy functions without sensible evacuations.

Alkali. A class of caustics.

Amenorrhœa. Suppression of the menses.

Anæsthetic. An agent that deprives of feeling.

Ammonia. An alkali.

Autopsy. Examination after death.

Antimony. A metal.

Antiphlogistic. Reducing ; cooling.

Astringent. Binding, contracting ; opposed to laxative.

Belladonna. A drug prepared from the deadly nightshade.

Bismuth. A metal.

Borax. A salt formed by a combination of boracic acid with soda.

Cantharides. Blistering plaster made of flies.

Caustic. A substance that when applied to flesh burns or corrodes.

Colchicum. A vegetable drug.

Cervix. The neck of the womb.

Chronic. Of long standing.

Citrate. Chemical drug, as citrate of iron.

Constipating. Crowding or cramming into a narrow compass.

Conservator. One who preserves from injury.

Conium. Poison hemlock.

Cupping. The operation of drawing blood with a cupping glass.

Cul-de-sac. A blind sack.

Cubeb. A vegetable drug.

Chlorosis. Green sickness, deficiency in blood.

Deplete. To bleed, to lower or weaken.

Diaphragm. The large breathing muscle between the chest and the belly.

Distended. Expanded.

Dietetic. Pertaining to food.

Displacement. Out of place.

Digitalis. The plant called foxglove.

Diuretic. Medicine that acts on the kidneys.

Drastic. Physicing; cathartic.

Dysmenorrhœa. Painful menstruation.

Elixir. A medicine.

Embryo. In physiology, the first rudiments of a new creature.

Emmenagogue. Medicine used to produce menstruation.

Emanation. Proceeding from.

Ergot. Blasted rye.

Fecal. Wastes discharged from the body.

Fistula. Pipe in ulcer, or narrow canal lined by false membrane.

Flatulence. Wind in stomach or bowels.

Fomentations. Hot applications.

Function. Office, action of an organ.

Germ. First principle.

Genital. Pertaining to the sexual.

Henbane. A poisonous plant.

Hepatic. Pertaining to the liver.

Hellebore. A poisonous plant.

Hemorrhage. Any discharge of blood from vessels destined to contain it.

Homeopathy. The doctrine that like cures like.

Hygienic. Healthful.

Hydrochloric. A drug used as a medicine.

Hysteralgia. A species of nervous affection.

Hygeio-Therapeutic. Treating diseases hygienically.

Inunction. To besmear, anoint.

Iodine. A medicine used as a local irritant.

Ipecac. A vegetable drug used as an emetic.

Jaundice. Disease of the liver.

Lacteal. Pertaining to milk.
Lavement. A washing or bathing, an injection.
Leech. A worm used in extracting blood.
Leucorrhœa. Discharge from uterus ; catarrh.
Logwood. Drug used in coloring.

Marasmus. Wasting.
Maltreatment. Bad treatment.
Magnesia. A drug, species of earth.
Menstrual. Pertaining to the menses.
Menorrhagia. Profuse menstruation, flooding.
Morbid. Not healthy, diseased.
Morphine. Preparation of opium.

Narcotic. Stupefying.
Nervine. Acting on the nervous system.
Neuralgia. Pain in a nerve.
Normal. Healthy.
Nosological. Pertaining to the classification of diseases.

Obstetric. Pertaining to midwifery.
Obstruction Hindrance, impediment.
Opprobrium medicorum. (Lat.) The reproach of physicians.
Organic. Pertaining to, or having, organs.
Ostracize. To cast out from social or private favor.
Oxygen. Air.

Pathology. Explains the nature and causes of disease.
Panada. A mixture of spirits and other ingredients for the
Pessary. A surgical instrument.   [sick.
Pelvic. Pertaining to the pelvis.
Pharmacopœa. A work which treats of drugs.
Physiology. Treats of functions.
Plethoric. Overfullness.
Protuberant. Protruding.
Prolapsus. Falling.
Prognosticate. To predict.
Puberty. The age at which a person is capable of begetting
    children.

Purgative. Physic.
Puerperal. Pertaining to childbirth.

Respiratory. The act of breathing.
Reproduction. To produce again.
Retroversion. Backward, falling back.
Rhubarb. A vegetable.
Rubefacient. A liniment.

Sacrum. Lower part of spine.
Savin. A drug.
Scarify. To cut.
Scrofulous. A constitutional disease.
Sedentary. Setting.
Secundem artem· According to rule.
Senega. Drug.
Seton. Rowel.
Sequelæ. (Lat.) Something that follows.
Sexual. Pertaining to sex.
Squills. Kind of onion used as a medicine.
Stamina. Force.
Sterility. Barrenness.
Strychnine. Medicine obtained from dog button.
Syncope. Fainting, or swooning.

Tannate. A compound of tannic acid and a base.
Technical. Specially appropriate.
Thorax. Pertaining to the chest.
Tonic. Giving tone.
Torpid. Inactive.
Toxicology. Doctrine of poisons.

Ultimatum. The last.
Umbilicus. The navel.
Uterus. The womb.

Vagina. A canal.
Veratrum. Drug.
Vertigo. Dizziness.
Viscera. Contents of the thorax, or abdomen.
Vital. Life.

OUR PLATFORM.

[At a meeting of the friends of Reform, held at the Health Reform Institute, Battle Creek, Mich., Jan. 1, 1872, this Platform was unanimously adopted.]

1. GOD, in the creation of man, established laws pertaining to both his moral and physical natures, which, had he always obeyed them, would have given him immunity from sickness, and would have perpetuated his life. Sickness and suffering had their origin in the violation of these laws.

2. As man cannot have eternal life without strict obedience to moral law, so he cannot have deliverance from the terrible bondage of sickness and premature death without strict observance of physical law.

3. The moral and physical natures of man are so intimately related that it is impossible to live in violation of either of these laws without doing violence to the other. Physical law, therefore, in its sphere, is as sacred and binding upon man as moral law.

4. The gospel teaches that man should live healthfully as well as righteously.

5. We recognize in nature the power to restore to health without the aid of medicines. The true physician supplies conditions : Nature cures.

6. Our *materia medica :* Good food, pure air, pure soft water, light, heat, exercise, proper clothing, rest, sleep, moral and social influences.

7. Our motto : Temperance in all things. Not only in eating, drinking, and in labor, but in everything that tends to exhaust the vitality of the system.

8. It has been well said, " A contented mind is a continual feast." A well-founded trust in God is the best and surest promoter of cheerfulness of mind ; and without this all other means may fail.

Health Reform Institute,

BATTLE CREEK, MICHIGAN.

THIS Institution has a competent corps of Physicians, both male and female, and is under the general supervision of a Board of Directors.

To those who are suffering from IMPAIRED HEALTH, and especially to those who have LOST CONFIDENCE IN DRUGS, we would say, *Do not Despair!* There is a method of treating disease, and of preserving health, so simple, and yet so efficient, that those who avail themselves of its benefits are saved an untold amount of suffering, and may escape an untimely grave. At this Institute diseases are treated on

HYGIENIC PRINCIPLES.

Instructions, both *Theoretical* and *Practical*, are given to Patients and Boarders on the great subject of

How to Live so as to Preserve Health,

and also respecting the safe and sure means of *Recovery from Disease.* In the treatment of the sick, No Drugs will be given. Those means only will be employed which NATURE CAN USE IN HER HEALING WORK; such as Proper Food, Water, Air, Light, Exercise, Cheerfulness, Rest, and Sleep.

GRAINS, VEGETABLES AND FRUITS,

CONSTITUTE THE STAPLE ARTICLES OF DIET.

This Institution is admirably located on a site of over seven acres, in the highest part of the pleasant and enterprising city of Battle Creek, commanding a fine prospect, and affording ample opportunities for entertainment, quiet, and retirement.

With a competent corps of PHYSICIANS and HELPERS, this Institution offers to the sick all the inducements to *Come and be Cured* that are presented by any other.

BATTLE CREEK is an important station on the Michigan Central and Peninsular Railroads, and is easy of access from all parts of the country.

ALL TRAINS STOP AT BATTLE CREEK.

☞ For Particulars see CIRCULAR, sent free on application.

Address **HEALTH INSTITUTE,** *Battle Creek, Mich.*

Kedzie's Water Filter.

THE KEDZIE IMPROVED WATER FILTER is one of the greatest and most useful inventions of the age.

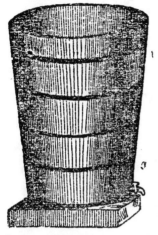 After years of labor and study, a Water Filter has been constructed so perfect in internal arrangements that every family or person having them in use are assured of pure, healthy water at all times; also know to a certainty that they are taking into the stomach no sort or kind of larvæ or spawn of worms,—or insects, or strange, loathsome animalculæ,—or impure floating matter that often lays the foundation of disease. This improved Reliable Water Filter readily removes all this; also, all gases, taste, color, or smell, from the water—consequently it must be pure, drinkable, and healthy.

Thousands use them; thousands praise them; thousands certify to their reliability and superior qualities over all others for perfectly purifying rain or river water, rendering it drinkable and healthy. The manufacturers are practical and scientific men, and understand perfectly the action of carbons, which enables them to produce the desired result.

This Kedzie Improved Water Filter is being sold throughout the United States and Canadas, and those who now have them in use certify to their utility, as a perfect purifier of water, and say to the manufacturers, "Make your Reliable Improved Filter generally known, for it works like a charm."

Manufactured by **R. A. BUNNEL,** Rochester, N. Y.

We furnish to order, **Kedzie's Water Filters,** at the following prices: No. 1, $9.00; No. 2, $10.50; No. 3, $12.00; No. 4, $13.50; No. 5, $15.00. Freight will be added.

Address **HEALTH REFORMER,** *Battle Creek, Mich*

HEALTH AND DISEASES

— OF —

WOMAN.

BY

R. T. TRALL, M. D.

Author of the "Hydropathic Encyclopedia;" "Hygienic Hand Book;"
"Uterine Diseases and Displacements;" "The True Healing
Art;" "True Temperance Platform; "Hygienic
System;" "Tobacco Using;" &c., &c.

PUBLISHED AT
THE OFFICE OF THE HEALTH REFORMER,
BATTLE CREEK, MICH.

THE HEALTH REFORMER.

AN APPEAL TO THE CANDID PUBLIC.

LADIES AND GENTLEMEN: Permit us to invite your attention to the *Health Reformer*, a monthly journal, devoted to the exposition of the laws of our being, and the application of those laws in the preservation of health and the treatment of disease.

The world is full of men and women who need reforming in their habits of life. And the present time, in some respects, is favorable to this work. As great changes in medical practice take place, the people lose confidence in drugs, and many of our public journals, which are circulating everywhere, speak of proper diet, bathing, exercise, and air, as the real reliances for health. Thus the superstitious confidence of people in doctors' doses is being shaken; the ice is broken, and the way prepared to spread abroad the true philosophy of life, health, and happiness.

The *Reformer* will avoid extreme positions, and will labor to disarm the people of their prejudice, and, in the spirit of love and good-will, appeal to them, and entreat them to turn from wrong habits of life, and live; and at the same time it will stand in independent defense of the broad principles of hygiene, and gather as many as possible upon this glorious platform.

And while the conductors of the *Reformer* may speak of God, Christ, the Holy Spirit, the Bible, and the Christian religion, in terms of reverence, they will studiously avoid giving this journal the least denominational cast. We more than welcome men and women of all religious denominations, and those who are not connected with any of the religious bodies, to all the benefits and blessings derived from correct habits of life.

Our journal will contain, each month, thirty-two pages of reading matter, from able and earnest pens, devoted to real, practical life, to physical, moral, and mental improvement. We design that each number shall contain articles upon Bi-

(See third page of cover.)

ble Hygiene. We take up the subject from the Sacred Record of the creation of man in Genesis, his employment, his surroundings in Eden, and the food given him of God, and trace the matter in the Scriptures of the Old and New Testaments.

With a large portion of the people, the Bible is the highest and safest authority in all matters of truth and duty. Prove to Christian men and women, who fear God and tremble at his word, that existing reformatory movements are in strict harmony with the teachings of the sacred Scriptures, and they will no longer regard the subject as unworthy of their notice. But the very general impression that the restrictions of the hygienic practice are not sustained by the word of God, has placed many sincere Christians where it is difficult to reach them.

And it is a painful fact that the vain philosophy, driveling skepticism, and the extremes of some who have been connected with the health-reform movement, have done much to prejudice sincere persons against the true philosophy of health. But those who revere God and his holy word can be reached with the plain declarations of the Scriptures of the Old and the New Testament. We promise to make it appear that the Bible does not justify Christians in many of the common and fashionable habits of our time, which sustain a close relation to life and health, but that it does demand of them changes from these wrong habits. If we succeed in doing this, it will be considered, by all Bible Christians, that it is highly proper that the attention of the Christian public should be called to the subject of Bible Hygiene, and that we may expect, so far as our journal is concerned, to receive liberal patronage from those who bear the Christian name.

Ladies and gentlemen, you need our journal, and we need your patronage. Please subscribe for it. It will cost you only the *small sum of one dollar a year.*

Address HEALTH REFORMER, *Battle Creek, Mich.*

OUR BOOK LIST.

The Hygienic System. By R. T. Trall, M. D. Recently published at the Office of the HEALTH REFORMER. It is just the work for the time, and should be read by the million. Price, post-paid, 20 cents.

The Health and Diseases of Woman. By R. T. Trall, M. D. A work of great value. Price, post-paid, 20 cents.

Tobacco-Using. A philosophical exposition of the Effects of Tobacco on the Human System. By R. T. Trall, M. D. Price, post-paid, 20 cents.

Cook Book. and Kitchen Guide: comprising recipes for the preparation of hygienic food, directions for canning fruit, &c., together with advice relative to change of diet. Price, post-paid, 20 cents.

Hydropathic Encyclopedia. Trall. Price, post-paid, $4.50.

Water Cure for the Million. Trall. Price, post-paid, 30 cents.

Uterine Diseases and Displacements. Trall. Price, post-paid, $3.00.

Science of Human Life. By Sylvester Graham, M. D. Price, post-paid, $3.00.

Valuable Pamphlet. Containing three of the most important of Graham's twenty-five Lectures on the Science of Human Life—eighth, the Organs and their Uses; thirteenth, Man's Physical Nature and the Structure of His Teeth; fourteenth, the Dietetic Character of Man. Price, post-paid, 35 cts.

Hydropathic Family Physician. By Joel Shew, M. D. Price, post-paid, $3.50.

Domestic Practice. Johnson. Price, post-paid, $1.75.

Hand Book of Health—Physiology and Hygiene. Published by the Health Reform Institute, Battle Creek, Mich. Price, post-paid, 75 cents; paper cover, 40 cents.

Water Cure in Chronic Diseases. By J. M. Gully, M. D. Price, post-paid, $1.75.

Cure of Consumption. Dr. Work. Price, post-paid, 30 cts.

Reform Tracts, by mail, in packages of not less than 200 pages, post-paid, at the rate of 800 pages for $1.00.

Address, **Health Reformer,** *Battle Creek, Mich.*